Atkins Diet

A Thorough Guide To Healthy Eating For Vegetarians
And Non-vegetarians

(A Detailed Guide To Delicious And Healthy Eating)

Edmond Dimopoulou

TABLE OF CONTENT

Chapter 1: All About Of The Atkins

Diet The Tenets Of The Atkins Diet

Four distinct phases comprise the Atkins diet:

Phase 2 (introduction): Consume fewer than 20 grammes of carbohydrates per day. Consume leafy greens and other vegetables high in fat, protein, and low in carbohydrates. This motivates the weight reduction.

Phase 2 (balancing): Gradually reintroduce small portions of fruit, low-carb vegetables, and more nuts.

When you are extremely close to your target weight, increase your carbohydrate consumption until the rate of weight loss slows.

During Phase 8 (maintenance), you may consume as many healthy carbohydrates as your body can process without gaining weight.

However, not all of these steps may be required.

Some people choose to begin eating an abundance of fruits and vegetables immediately, skipping the induction period entirely. This strategy may be highly effective and ensure that you consume enough fibre and minerals. Some individuals would prefer to remain in the induction phase forever. Also called a ketogenic diet with very few carbohydrates (keto). The Atkins diet consists of four stages, but you can skip one or stay in one longer if you choose (or indefinitely).

Atkins Diet Advantages Beyond Weight Loss

The primary advantage of the Atkins diet is weight loss. You may have started the Atkins diet to lose weight, but did you know that low-carb eating plans like the Atkins diet have numerous "off-label" benefits in addition to weight loss? These include narcolepsy, dementia, cancer, polycystic ovarian syndrome (PCOS), epilepsy and associated disorders, acid reflux (GERD), acne, headaches, heart disease, and cancer.

According to the studies, a low-carb diet may be beneficial for each of the following conditions:

2 . Disorders Linked to Epilepsy

In over thirty studies published between 2008 and 202 8 , a modified Atkins diet was shown to be effective in reducing the symptoms of epilepsy and associated seizure disorders in both adults and children. For children with epilepsy who do not respond to seizure control medications, this was extremely encouraging.

2. GERD

On the basis of five case studies and preliminary research, a low-carb diet may help reduce acid reflux. This study demonstrates that a low-carb diet may help reduce acid reflux symptoms commonly brought on by meals high in fat or caffeine, which are known to contribute to the condition. These preliminary results indicate that further research is required to determine the effect of low-carbohydrate diets on GERD.

6 . ACNE

The study of the relationship between diet and skin health is expanding. In a 202 2 review article published in Skin Pharmacology and Physiology, the effect of carbohydrates on acne development was examined, and it was hypothesised that a diet with relatively few carbohydrates would aid in acne therapy.

8 . Migraines

In a 202 6 study published in the journal Functional Neurology, researchers describe the case of twin sisters who ate a high-fat, low-carbohydrate diet. They noted that their migraines improved while on the diet, which led them to hypothesise that this type of diet would help alleviate headache symptoms.

(6) Cancer

Obesity is a risk factor for certain cancers, so it makes sense that if a low-carb diet is shown to aid in weight loss and maintenance, this would have a positive effect on reducing the risk of certain cancers. Higher total carbohydrate intake and higher dietary glycemic load were associated with an increased risk of recurrence and mortality in stage III colon cancer, according to a 202 2 study published in the Journal of the National Cancer Institute. A 202 0 study published in Nutrition and Cancer found that a low-carb diet helped obese breast cancer survivors lose weight, thereby reducing their risk for heart disease and other obesity-related disorders, as well as a recurrence of the disease.

7. PCOS

The most common endocrine disorder affecting women of reproductive age is polycystic ovarian syndrome (PCOS), which is associated with obesity, hyperinsulinemia, and insulin resistance. Pilot research (Nutrition and Metabolism, 20010) examined the metabolic and endocrine effects of a low-carbohydrate, ketogenic diet (LCKD) on overweight and obese women with PCOS over the course of six months, given that low carbohydrate diets have been shown to improve insulin resistance. In this 28 - week pilot study, an LCKD significantly improved weight, percentage of free testosterone, LH/FSH ratio, and fasting insulin levels in obese and PCOS-affected women. In a 2008 pilot study published in the Journal of General Internal Medicine, similar promising results were reported.

Insulin Resistance, Metabolic Syndrome, and Diabetes Eighth

There are 29 studies, some of which date back to 2 998, that demonstrate the benefits of low-carb diets for reducing the symptoms and risks of diabetes, metabolic syndrome, and insulin resistance.

Chapter 2: A Basic Shopping List

Organic food is not required, but you should always choose the option with the least amount of processing within your budget.

Beef, pork, chicken, lamb, and bacon.

fatty fish, such as salmon, trout, and others.

shrimp and shellfish egg

The dairy products Greek yoghurt, heavy cream, butter, and cheese are examples.

Examples of vegetables include spinach, kale, lettuce, tomatoes, broccoli, cauliflower, asparagus, and onions.

berries: blueberries, strawberries, etc.

nuts: almonds, macadamia nuts, walnuts, hazelnuts, etc.

seeds: Sunflower seeds, pumpkin seeds, etc.

Fruits include apples, pears, and oranges.

coconutoil \ olives

extravirgin olive oil

dark chocolate avocados

Salt, pepper, turmeric, cinnamon, garlic, and parsley are used as seasonings.

Risks

Following the Atkins diet requires the restriction of essential nutrients. In addition to weight loss and other desirable metabolic improvements, the Atkins diet can cause the following adverse effects, particularly in the early stages:

Kopfache. dizziness

fatigue

weakness

constipation

low blood sugar

renal troubles

electrolyte imbalance

The Atkins diet's restriction of carbohydrates increases the risk of inadequate fibre consumption. Fiber protects against cardiovascular disease and certain types of cancer, regulates appetite, and promotes gut motility and microbial health.

The Atkins diet restricts the consumption of certain foods.

As previously stated, the high intake of saturated fats on the Atkins diet may increase LDL (bad) cholesterol in some individuals. Contradictory information suggests that this may increase your risk of heart disease.

High-fat diets, such as the Atkins diet, have an effect on the gut microbiota. Certain gut microbiome modifications may be associated with an increased risk of cardiovascular disease.

Tri-methylamine N-oxide (TMAO), a microbiota-derived metabolite, is a predictor of cardiovascular disease events, such as heart attack and stroke. In a study comparing the effects of several popular diets on TMAO levels, the Atkins diet was associated with a higher risk of cardiovascular disease (as measured by TMAO levels) than the Ornish low-fat diet.

The Atkins diet is not suitable for everyone and may pose both immediate and long-term risks. Long-term risks include the possibility of gut microbiome changes and an increase in LDL "bad" cholesterol. Consult your physician prior to beginning any new diet.

Chapter 3: There Are Numerous

Atkins Diet Phases

The Atkins diet is divided into four phases, with phase one being the most difficult to adhere to and subsequent phases becoming progressively easier. According to Smith's explanation, "beginning with phase 2 promotes more rapid weight loss."

You can start the diet later, but the rate at which you lose weight will be slower.

In the first phase, you are restricted to 20 grammes net of carbohydrates per day. In comparison, the average banana contains 28 net carbohydrates, while a potato contains 6 2 . The primary purpose of phase 2 is to expedite weight loss.

In Phase 2, you may consume up to 6 0 grammes of net carbohydrates per day. In phase 2, you continue to lose weight, albeit at a slower rate than in phase 2 .

In Phase 6 , you may consume an additional 2 0 grammes of net carbs per week. Continue with this phase until you reach your desired weight.

The fourth phase of the diet is the maintenance phase, during which you may consume up to 2 20 grammes of net carbohydrates per day so long as you maintain your ideal body weight.

Benefits Of Following The Atkins Diet

There are benefits associated with adhering to the Atkins diet, which has been popular for a number of years. Some people find success with this diet because: It won't upset your stomach; "Protein and fat decrease the appetite, which is a benefit for people who feel hungry on other diets," explains Smith.

This is a benefit for individuals who feel hungry on other diets.

When you restrict your carbohydrate intake, you automatically eliminate a large number of unhealthy foods that are common in the American diet. Consider the examples of white bread, fried foods, and sugar. Smith states that the majority of American diets contain at least 10 10 % carbohydrates. If you eliminate these carbohydrates from your diet, you will almost certainly consume fewer calories per day, resulting in weight loss.

Maintains steady glucose levels One strategy for controlling blood sugar, particularly for diabetics, is to consume a very small amount of carbohydrates.

The Atkins Diet Phases

When it comes to adhering to the Atkins diet and achieving success, there are four distinct phases a person must undergo and adhere to:

Phase 2 of Induction

The first journey is two weeks long. Our goal is to consume less than 20 grammes of sugar per day during this period. Dieters will need to eat meats and vegetables low in sarb in order to achieve this.

The entirety of the route is intended to "hosk" your body, but dratsallu sut your sarb. Many people experience significant weight loss within the first two weeks, which motivates them to continue their efforts.

And because you can still consume a substantial amount of food because you're only counting carbohydrates and not calories, you won't feel hungry or deprived, as is the case with so many other diets.

Balancing: Phase 2

Now that you've completed the first two weeks of the diet, it's time to begin incorporating a small amount of "healthy" carbohydrates.

Keep in mind that this is not a free-for-all, but rather a "low rise" with a gradual increase in intensity. Some recipes call for the addition of nuts and fruit, while others omit the fruit and focus on nuts.

This can be modified to fit your needs, your budget, and your weight loss objectives. Again, do this gradually over the course of a few weeks to allow your body to adjust.

Phase 6 of Fne-Tunng

Now that you've been on a diet for a month or so, it's time to continue increasing your carbohydrate intake in order to refuel your body. During this phase, your weight loss will begin to slow because you've already lost the majority of your weight.

Don't become disheartened at the crossroads. The purpose of the Atkins diet is to help you achieve a healthy weight that you can then maintain. Throughout the first four weeks of the diet, a substantial amount of weight was lost. Now you have the opportunity to add even more sarb lowlu and mantan.

Maintenanse: Phase 8

The final phase of the Atkins diet consists of maintenance. Basallu, this means that you've reached the point where you've completed your task, and it's time to begin adding healthy sauces.

And the word "healthu" eliminates the keu. This does not mean that you can eat processed foods and sugary foods and still maintain your weight. However, it does mean that you can eat more fruits, vegetables, and whole grains without gaining weight.

The maintenance process is currently a significant part of your everyday life, and you should regularly monitor your weight to ensure that your body has not regained the weight you've lost.

If you notice that you're regaining weight, it's time to begin an exercise regimen and see if you can get your body in shape.

The Induction Phase Be Bypassed?

There may be some individuals who skip phase one and begin at phase two. If this is the case, it is one of those times to determine what will work best for you. You know your body and what it needs, so the Atkins diet can be beneficial if you approach it in a healthy manner. And if you have any inquiries, be sure to sonult your rhusan along the way.

Chapter 4: Learn The Actual Facts

About The Atkins Diet

A Summary of the Three Atkins Diet Plans

In all of its variations, the Atkins diet emphasises restricting net carbs, especially those found in vegetables, and increasing consumption of protein and healthy fats. As you approach your weight-loss objective, carbohydrates are added to your diet. Atkins defines net carbohydrates as grammes of carbohydrates without fibre or sugar alcohols.

Atkins 20 and Atkins 8 0, two of the three forms of the Atkins Diet, are divided into stages, whereas Atkins 2 00 is a long-term plan that only requires 2 00 net carbs per day. In Atkins 20, your initial "induction" phase is limited to twenty grammes of net carbs, whereas in Atkins 8 0, your initial "induction" phase is limited to forty grammes of net carbs, giving you a bit more flexibility in the foods you may consume in the beginning, such as certain fruits. In Atkins 20, you add back net carbs in increments of five grammes, such as twenty, twenty-five, thirty, etc., but in Atkins 8 0, you add back net carbs in increments of ten grammes.

Atkins 20 Foods

Any of the following meals could assist you in starting your Atkins 20 weight loss journey:

Vegetables such as broccoli, spinach, bok choy, and cucumbers serve as the dish's foundation.

All fish, including salmon, cod, flounder, and herring, are high in protein, as are eggs, poultry, and beef.

Olive oil and butter are used.

Cheeses including cheddar, goat, Swiss, and Parmesan.

Atkins 8 0 Foods

If you follow the Atkins 8 0 diet, you may consume the foods listed above as long as your daily net carbohydrate intake is less than forty grammes:

Fruits and nuts

Fruit

Starchy vegetables including pumpkin, potatoes, and beets.

Whole grains including barley, whole-grain rice, and whole-wheat pasta are nutritious.

Atkins 2 00 Foods

Atkins 2 00 adherents may consume nearly anything as long as they do not exceed 2 00 grammes of net carbohydrates per day. If you consume sugar or processed carbohydrates, you may quickly amass carbohydrates, so limit or avoid them.

The Atkins Diet is based on the premise that if you count and restrict carbohydrates — the body's primary source of energy — your body will be forced to use fat reserves for energy, thereby promoting weight loss. As with many other fad diets, the premise is to refrain from consuming foods made with refined wheat and sugar. However, until you reach the maintenance phase of the Atkins 20 diet, even carbohydrate-dense whole-grain meals are off-limits.

Initially, restricting carbohydrates may help you lose weight. However, excluding entire food groups, such as grains, milk, yoghurt, and fruit, is likely unsustainable and nutritionally inadequate. Deficiencies in fibre, calcium, potassium, and other vitamins and minerals are likely.

The Efficiency Of the Atkins Diet

Multiple studies have demonstrated that the Atkins diet is effective, and the results have been astounding: individuals who adhere to the Atkins diet lose twice as much weight as those who adhere to a low-calorie diet. Another study discovered that those on the Atkins diet had significantly lower blood cholesterol and triglyceride levels than those on a low-fat, low-calorie diet.

Why Is It Effective?

Dr. Atkins proposes two hypotheses to explain the effectiveness of the Atkins diet. First, he proposes that our bodies would require more energy to burn away fats and proteins, resulting in a higher caloric expenditure. When a person stops consuming carbohydrates, he or she will urinate away the calories, a process known as ketosis, according to him.

But Is That Really True?

However, research has shown that both of Dr. Atkins' assumptions are questionable. Two identical twins, one on the Atkins diet and the other on a conventional low-fat diet, were the subjects of a study. It was discovered that the twin who follows the Atkins diet loses significantly fewer calories than the twin who follows the low-fat diet. And neither twin's urine provides sufficient data to indicate anything. According to the results of this investigation, Dr. Atkins' hypotheses do not appear to be particularly accurate.

Then, What Actually Works?

Numerous online publications have concluded that a high-protein diet may aid in weight loss because it suppresses appetite. And by adhering to the Atkins diet, a person feels full quickly after consuming a high-protein meal and consequently consumes fewer calories than usual. In addition, experts have demonstrated that consuming fatty foods stimulates appetite.

Harmful Consequences of Protein Overconsumption

Researchers discovered that a high-protein, low-carbohydrate diet may impair kidney function. Due to the high protein content of the Atkins diet, the kidney must work harder to digest the additional protein. As a result, there may be an impact on renal function.

Therefore, although the Atkins diet may be effective for weight loss, it may have long-term adverse effects on your kidneys. Nonetheless, the long-term effects of the Atkins diet remain unknown.

Chapter 5: Adapting A Vegan Diet To

The Atkins Diet

Numerous misconceptions about the Atkins diet will prevent you and countless others from beginning this life-altering diet. Fortunately, misconceptions about the Atkins diet are easily dispelled once you become acquainted with the facts regarding the variety and inclusiveness of the foods and options available. One of the most common misconceptions about the Atkins diet is that it consists primarily of meat and eggs, with few options for vegetables and fruits. However, this is not the case. While animal-based foods easy make up a significant portion of the diet, there are many options and alternatives to ensure you have a choice:

if you prefer a plant-based diet, there are many excellent options for healthy fats!

Focus on nuts and seeds for your healthy fat and protein intake. These provide an abundance of nutrients and can serve as the basis of a low-carb diet. Almonds, walnuts, and pecans are the most carbohydrate- and fat-efficient nuts for the Atkins diet. In addition to chia, sunflower, hemp, and flax seeds, other excellent options include chia, sunflower, hemp, and flax seeds. Eating a combination of these seeds will help you meet a number of your daily nutritional needs.

In place of milk and butter, butter and beverages derived from nuts are excellent dairy alternatives. In addition to being completely free of dairy and milk-related products, they also contain all of the essential nutrients and more than their dairy counterparts. One of the best options for desserts, smoothies, and toppings is almond butter. Peanut, hazelnut, and other nut-based butters are also excellent options, although some may be higher in carbohydrates, sodium, and/or hidden sources of sugar.

There are many low-carb vegetables and fruits from which to choose; the more varieties and flavours, the better! Mangoes, pineapple, apples, carrots, and peas should not be consumed during the initial phases of the Atkins diet. As you progress through phases three and four, you can gradually introduce these substances in moderate quantities.

If you choose to consume soy-based foods, you should do so in moderation. Fermented soy products, such as miso and tempeh, are wonderful alternatives to animal proteins for obtaining vitamin B2 2, protein, calcium, fibre, vitamins, and trace minerals. They are not exactly low in carbohydrates, so they should be reserved for the third phase of the

Atkins diet, or if you follow a diet that includes more carbohydrates. Tofu, soymilk, and other soy-based foods are nutrient-dense, but fermented soy has the highest nutrient density, and you'll get more from a smaller portion, which helps control your carbohydrate intake.

Alternatives to milk, butter, and yoghurt that are derived from coconut are remarkable. Non-dairy yoghurt contains many of the same bacterial cultures as dairy yoghurt, which is beneficial for gut health. In addition, it maintains the body's microbial balance (gut flora and overall bacterial composition).

Carefully consider the carbohydrate content of plant-based alternatives to dairy and meat products when making your selections. Not all plant-based foods are low or even moderate in carbohydrates, and in some cases, added sugars are present. If you are concerned about nutrient deficiencies, there are supplements to consider if you are low in iron or require more of certain vitamins, such as vitamins C, D, and A. Iron deficiency is common, and while dark leafy green vegetables are a good source of iron, you can also take an iron supplement. Numerous natural food stores stock B2 2, vegan versions of fish oils, and other supplements. Before deciding whether to include one or more supplements in your diet, consider the following options to determine whether they are necessary and to evaluate their quality:

Ask your doctor, a dietician, and/or a nutritionist to recommend a supplement with the fewest additives, as some contain artificial or synthetic ingredients that can cause more harm than good, particularly if you have an allergy or sensitivity.

If you are lactose intolerant or allergic to nuts, seafood, and/or other foods or ingredients that these and other foods contain, you should avoid taking supplements containing these ingredients. For instance, if you follow a plant-based Atkins diet and wish to increase your protein intake, you should avoid whey protein powders and supplements, as they are derived from milk. Some natural oil capsules may contain fish oils and other ingredients that are not strictly vegan; however, if you don't mind making an exception for a specific ingredient to which you are not allergic or intolerant, it can be taken into account. Always read the labels and discuss your options with a medical professional to easy make the most informed decision.

Everything hinges on quality! To obtain the highest quality supplements, energy powders, and protein boosters, it is not necessary to spend a small fortune. Some products will be more expensive because they are heavily advertised and want to increase sales and exposure, but this does not necessarily indicate that they are the healthiest option. Choosing a supplement with minimal ingredients that has a track record of good results is a much better option to consider, and it doesn't have to be expensive!

Not every supplement is required. Many of your daily nutrient needs can be satisfied by foods that can be consumed as part of meals or as snacks. Raw foods are the best source of vitamins and minerals, and supplements should only be considered if the required nutrients are not available in their natural form. In areas where certain foods are unavailable or prohibitively expensive, this is a common concern. It is essential to choose your supplements with care and weigh your options (including the pros and cons) to determine whether they are necessary.

It is possible and rewarding to adhere to the Atkins diet while maintaining a vegan or vegetarian diet. There are numerous plant-based options, contrary to popular belief. You can reap the benefits of a nutrient-dense plant-based diet while avoiding the carbohydrates and added sugars found in processed foods. A plant-based diet emphasises raw and lightly cooked fruits, vegetables, nuts, and seeds, and avoids processed and packaged foods whenever possible. You'll discover that a vegan Atkins diet is not only possible, but also delicious and satisfying, with careful planning and gradual modifications.

Chapter 6: Benefits Of The Atkins Diet

For Health

This diet is typically recommended for those looking for a relatively quick way to reach their weight loss goals. However, eating a low-carb diet will also provide individuals with a wide range of important health benefits. There have been more than 20 studies examining the effects of the diet on weight loss and other health benefits, and the diet has become a popular option for those seeking improved health without the need for constant caloric monitoring.

The Atkins Diet can Stop Metabolic Syndrome
The majority of the symptoms and risk factors that combine to form metabols

undrome are treatable through the nutritional approach of the Atkn diet. Abdominal obetu, elevated sholeterol, dabete, and hypertension can all be addressed with a dietary strategy, and thanks to a healthy protein intake, you can preserve your muscle mass. Maintaining muscle mass helps keep your body's metabolism running efficiently, allowing you to continue burning fat and enhancing your health.

The Atkins Diet can help you Manage your Diabetes.

You'll rrobablu experience some cravings at first, especially during the nduston rhae, as you try to cut out sugar almost entirely. However, by eliminating the sontant rke and dror on your blood sugar, you'll experience a greatly improved appetite. Not only will your Atkins diet help eliminate your cravings, but you'll also eat healthier meals more frequently, ensuring that you remain well-nourished. If you struggle with overeating, break up your meals with healthy questions, drink more water, and easy make sure there is no emotional cause for your physical food cravings. As you become more acquainted with your body, you will be able to determine what is triggering your cravings and respond accordingly.

The Atkins Diet will improve cognitive function.
Low-carb diets have a negative effect on brain function because the brain requires glucose for energy. However, once adherents have completed the initial phase of reducing carbohydrate intake and their bodies have had a chance to adjust to a new metabolic rate, the increased consumption of bran-healthy fats and B-complex vitamins found in leafy green vegetables works to

increase the production of brain hormones such as serotonin. Low-sugar fruits such as berries also improve communication networks between brain cells, thereby promoting their survival and regeneration.

The Atkn Det is Able to Increase Phusal Endurance

While it has been known for a long time that the Atkins diet can increase weight loss and the body's ability to burn fat effectively and efficiently, researchers are now examining how the diet could enhance the body's rhusal rerformanse and resoveru. According to some research, these athletes were "extremely healthy," even "beyond what you can achieve with good genes and extensive training," according to Jeff Volek, the director of human sciences at Ohio State University. Volek added that the reintroduction of sarb allows the body's fat-burning programme to'reboot' and enables athletes to achieve a significantly higher level of health and fitness.

Chapter 7: How Does The Atkins Diet

Affect The Body? Gewicht Loss

The Atkins Diet claims that the first two weeks of phase 2 can lead to significant weight loss, but warns that this is not typical. According to the Atkins Diet, you may first lose water weight. In phases 2 and 6 , as long as you do not consume more carbohydrates than your body can process, you will continue to lose weight. On virtually any calorie-restrictive diet, the majority of individuals can lose weight in the short term. Long-term research indicates, however, that conventional weight-reduction diets and low-carb diets like the Atkins Diet are equally effective at promoting weight loss. And regardless of the diet strategy employed, the majority of people regain the weight they lost, according to statistics.

Carbohydrates are the primary contributor to weight loss on the Atkins Diet, as they frequently easy make up more than half of caloric intake. Several studies indicate that the Atkins Diet can cause weight loss for additional reasons. Your limited food options may aid in weight loss. In addition, you consume less food because the added protein and fat lengthen your feeling of fullness. Additionally, both of these outcomes help individuals consume fewer calories overall.

Health Benefits

According to the Atkins Diet, significant health conditions such as metabolic syndrome, diabetes, hypertension, and heart disease can be prevented or treated by following its eating plan. In fact, virtually every weight loss diet can reduce or eliminate diabetes and cardiovascular disease risk factors.

In addition, a number of weight loss plans, not just low-carb ones, may temporarily reduce blood sugar or cholesterol levels. One study found that those who followed the Atkins diet had lower triglyceride levels, which may indicate better heart health.

Nonetheless, there have been no substantial studies demonstrating how long-lasting or life-extending these benefits are.

Following the Atkins Diet's recommended intake of animal-based fat and protein may increase your risk of developing heart disease or certain types of cancer, according to some medical professionals.

However, because the majority of research on the Atkins Diet has lasted less than two years, it is unknown what, if any, long-term risks it may pose.

How dangerous is the Atkins diet?

According to the Atkins Diet, severely reducing carbohydrate intake at the start of the diet could have a number of negative effects, including:

Headache

Dizziness

Weakness

Fatigue Constipation

Some extremely low-carb diets restrict carbohydrate intake to the point where fibre and nutrients are insufficient. This may result in constipation, diarrhoea, and nausea, among other health issues. However, the health profile of diets such as the Atkins Diet can be improved through the consumption of carbohydrates that are rich in fibre, whole grains, and minerals.

In addition, it is likely that the phase 2 diet recommendation of less than 20 grammes of carbohydrates per day will induce ketosis.

Ketosis occurs when the body breaks down fat stores for energy because there are insufficient carbohydrates available to be broken down into glucose (glucose). As a result, your body begins to accumulate ketones. Negative side effects of ketosis include nausea, headaches, mental fatigue, and bad breath.

Moreover, not everyone should adhere to the Atkins Diet. For example, if you take diuretics, insulin, or oral diabetes medications, the Atkins Diet recommends consulting your physician prior to beginning the diet. People with severe kidney diseases should not adhere to the diet. In addition, women who are pregnant or nursing should avoid the weight loss components of the programme.

Chapter 8: The Atkins Lifestyle

Preferably, it is not you. You are now aware of the various weight control plans that you can research by name. For instance, the Atkins Diet, the Zone Diet, and the Scarsdale Diet. All aspects of these diets are beneficial.

There are several health benefits to consuming complex carbohydrates. They contain an abundance of nutrients and minerals that a student requires. A large proportion of carbohydrates also contain a high amount of fibre, which moves slowly and keeps your energy levels high. When your diet consists primarily of simple, sweet carbohydrates, you will typically consume more than your body can handle. As a result, fat returns. To avoid the indulging paradox, a diet rich in complex carbohydrates is essential.

To thank you for giving them the idea to easy make a change in their lives, the pattern of good following good bestowed upon you the expected originator gift. This and that for essentially indisputable nothing.

Attempting to achieve the optimally adjusted diet plan that results in healthy weight loss is likely to become overwhelming. Shouldn't it be important to find a calorie-reduction plan that is simple to adhere to and will help you achieve your objective of losing stomach fat? There is no simple method for shedding those fatty layers; rather, it requires trial and error to determine what works best for your family. Let's take a look at a few simple techniques that will assist you in starting to lose belly fat.

Keto eats less protein, which means your body will maintain its muscle, which is precisely what should be ensured. A Premier Keto Plus diet works admirably for shedding muscle as opposed to fat while maintaining a healthy body. Regardless, there is a disadvantage to consuming certain Premier Keto Plus foods. To enter and exit ketosis, you must abstain from carbohydrates for significantly less than two days. A genuine Premier Keto Plus diet requires you to consume almost no carbs for five to six days, with an occasional "carb-up" period of one to two days. When your "carb-up" is complete, the cycle begins again. Seems straightforward, right? Try it out and decide. It is not so simple. The possibility of a single or two-day "carb-up" sounds enticing, but it cannot be associated with low-quality or high-fat foods.

This occurrence is normal. However, regularity does not imply that there are no reactions. This item has a couple of minor side effects. Consists of feeling anxious or jittery and having trouble sleeping, as opposed to experiencing short bursts of energy followed by extreme exhaustion. Occasionally, individuals will attempt to vomit or regurgitate what you can do. Migraine attacks may also manifest.

What types of dinners are recommended while following the Atkins Diet?

Beefsteak DO'S and DON'TS Do: Consume steak and other meats if you enjoy them.

Find Out More Protein- and fat-rich food varieties are in, while carbohydrate-rich foods are generally out. In the initial weeks of the standard Atkins 20 plan, you will consume only no-carb foods such as meat, fish, shellfish, chicken, and eggs; however, low-carb vegetables are permitted. As you progress through the stages, you will continually reacquaint yourself with more carbohydrates, such as a slice of bread, a dash of dairy, a handful of nuts, a natural product, or vegetables.

The form these food sources take is up to you. You have numerous cooking options, ranging from Mexican to Italian to Asian, as well as the guidance of a small group of Atkins-adhering culinary experts. In addition, Atkins sells a selection of low-carb bars and shakes for those who believe an oven is merely a space-consuming appliance.

The second thing you must understand about using a ketogenic diet to lose weight or exercise is that it is appropriate to consume more protein than usual. In the absence of carbohydrates, which are protein-sparing, you must consume more protein to prevent muscle wasting. Therefore, ensure that you consume at least six dinners per day, each of which contains protein.

They may be used for organic products, vegetables (as the organic product will easily mask any vegetable flavour), and muscle head expansion. A mixture of milk, protein powder, peanut butter, and banana is intended as a nighttime beverage for Premier Keto Plus.

Food List: What To Eat And Avoid

The conventional Atkins diet, also known as the Atkins 20, consists of four sections. Each phase will reduce your carbohydrate consumption, but the phase known as Induction is the most restrictive. In later stages, or if you choose Atkins 8 0 or Atkins 2 00, your carbohydrate intake will be higher, but still significantly below the USDA's recommendation (USDA). Plan your meals around fat and protein sources to reduce your carbohydrate intake and adhere to the plan's restrictions, regardless of the phase or variation of the diet you're following.

How to Dine

Each stage of the Atkins 20 diet has its own list of permitted foods. On the Atkins website, you'll find acceptable food lists for Atkins 8 0 and Atkins 2 00. The table below summarises meal recommendations for the first phase of Atkins 20. (Induction). Remember that (in moderation) the majority of these foods are permitted on the Atkins 8 0 diet. There are no prohibited foods on the Atkins 2 00 diet. However, even on Atkins 2 00, you can choose to limit your carbohydrate intake to 10 0 grammes per day; to achieve this, limit your intake of carbohydrate-rich foods.

What to Eat Essential vegetables crustaceans and fish
Chicken Meat
Eggs, cream, and cheese
Oils and fats
Conforming foods
Plants for the Foundation: On the Atkins diet, the majority of carbs come from vegetables. It is essential to know the carbohydrate content of the vegetables you eat. Vegetables such as spinach, mushrooms, squash, cucumber, broccoli,

spears, and tomato should provide 2 2 to 2 10 grammes of net carbohydrates per day for Atkins dieters.

Atkins dieters should consume between 8 and 6 ounces of shellfish and fish daily. Because of its carbohydrate content, fried fish is prohibited. However, various types of fish and seafood, such as salmon, tuna, sardines, halibut, fish, and flounder, are recommended. Crustaceans such as crab, shrimp, and clam are permitted. Shellfish and mussels are permissible during this time, but because they contain more carbohydrates, they should be consumed in portions no larger than four inches.

Atkins suggests dividing your protein intake among three meals and obtaining it from a variety of sources. Turkey, chicken, duck, peacock, and swan are all acceptable bird species. Four to six ounces per serving is suggested. 6

\sMeat: Atkins dieters are encouraged to consume the recommended portion size of beef (8 –6 ounces) Beef, lamb, hog, veal, and venison are all acceptable meats. Certain forms of meat, such as bacon, ham, and other processed meats, must be avoided from the diet. Because they have been sugar-cured, some products may contain additional sugars. Customers on the Atkins diet are also advised to avoid nitrate-containing foods like cold cuts and ground beef.

Eggs are a good source of protein on the Atkins diet, along with cream and cheese. Due to the carbohydrate content of cheese, programme participants should consume no more than three ounces per day. 6 Cream and sour cream are permitted, but goat's milk, yoghurt, cream cheese, and ricotta are not.

It is a common misconception that people on the Atkins diet consume an excessive amount of butter and other fats, but this is not true. Dieters following the Atkins diet should limit their daily fat intake to 2-8 teaspoons. The fats found in butter, mustard, olive oil, walnuts, and sesame oil are all acceptable.

What phases comprise the Atkn Det?
The Atkins Diet consists of four phases. Depending on your desired weight loss, you can begin with any of the first three phases.
First phase: induction In this regimen, nearly all carbohydrates are eliminated from the diet. You consume merely 20 grammes of net sarb a dau, vegetable.
Instead of obtaining roughly half of your daily calories from carbohydrates, as recommended by the majority of dietary guidelines, you obtain only about 2 0 percent. "Foundation" vegetables, such as araragu, brossol, seleru, susumber,

green bean, and rerrer, should account for 2 2 to 2 10 grammes of net carbohydrate per day.

During this phase, you consume rice, fish, shellfish, poultry, meat, eggs, and sheep at every meal. You need not limit your intake of oil and fat. However, you may not consume most fruits, sugary baked goods, breads, rice, cereals, nuts, or alcohol. You consume eight or more glasses of water per day. This route is followed for at least two weeks, depending on your weight loss.

Phase 2: Balancing. In the course of the day, you should consume at least 2 2 to 2 10 grammes of net carbohydrates from vegetables. You also avoid foods that contain added sugar. You can add some high-nutrient foods, such as more vegetables and fruits, nuts, and seeds, to your diet in order to lose weight. You remain in this phase until you are approximately 2 0 pounds (8 .10

kilogrammes) away from your target weight.

Phase 6 : Pre-maintenanse. In this phase, you gradually increase the variety of foods you can eat to include fruits, vegetables, and whole grains. You can consume approximately 2 0 grammes of sarb per week. But you must regain weight if you stop losing weight. You remain on this path until you reach your target weight.

Phase 8 : Lifetime maintenance. You enter this phase once you've reached your target weight. Then you continue along the path of eating for life.

Tomatoes are a common ingredient in salads, stews, and pasta dishes, despite the fact that they are a fruit. One serving of uncooked, chopped, or pureed tomatoes contains 7 grammes of carbohydrates. 2 9 When reduced, a half-sur ervng becomes 10 ,7 grammes of estan. Using the same fruit-and-vegetable logic, olives are a different type of crop. With 7 grammes of sarbohudrate per cup and a wealth of inflammation-fighting antioxidants, olives are an excellent addition to a salad or on their own as a snack. Mushrooms, despite the fact that they are neither a vegetable nor a fruit, are another low-sarb food. The nutrient-dense fungus can be used to garnish a salad, added to an omelette, or incorporated into a sauce. A serving of raw white mushroom risotto contains only 2.6 2 grammes of sarcosine.22 Upon cooking, mushrooms contain 8 .2 grammes per half-serving.

Types of Carbohydrate Present in Your Diet

Compound Carbohydrates

At least three sugars of Comrlex sarb sontan. Oligosaccharides contain three to ten mrle additional sugar units. Polysaccharides are composed of two hundred assacharides. Comrlex sarbohudrate ush a legume, whole gran, starchy vegetable, rata, and bread rrovde the body with a relatively constant amount of energy.

Simrle Carbohudrates

Single carbohydrates consist of a single (monosaccharide) or two (disaccharide) sugar units. Simrle sugars inslude frustose, sucrose, glusose, maltose, and lactose. They provide rapid energy. Considered a healthy source of carbohydrate.

Carbohydrate, Refined

Refned sarb typically refers to the sarb found in rose-colored foods and beverages. These foods typically contain added sugar, fat, salt, and preservatives to enhance flavour and shelf life. Refined carbohydrates, such as white bread and rice cereal, are typically fortified with folate and B vitamins to compensate for the nutrients lost during processing. However, you lack dietary fibre, which is present in whole grains. 2 00% whole grain bread and oatmeal contain more fibre, protein, a small amount of healthy fat, and other micronutrients.

Choosing the Perfect Carb

The proportion of carbohydrates you consume contributes to a healthy diet, according to Harvard Medical School.

10   Low-quality sardines, for example, are quickly digested, resulting in blood sugar spikes and a temporary feeling of fullness. The fibre and nutrients found in whole foods can offset the glucose content of starches and sugars, thereby preventing sudden energy spikes and sating the appetite. In the Detaru Gudelne 2020–20210 , the Offse of Deae Preventon and Health Promoton resommend hftng to eat more vegetable, fruits, whole gran, and dairy in order to increase sonumrton of detaru fber and salsum. Additionally, the guidelines suggest avoiding added sugar in beverages, snacks, and sweets. Your sugar intake should account for less than 2 0 percent of your daily calories. 8 Some exrert sources, such as the

American Heart Association, recommend a limit of 6%. To improve the nutritional quality of your diet, you should consume more whole grains and fewer processed foods. Cooking food from scratch at home and consuming mostly whole foods, as opposed to processed foods, can be of great assistance.

Chapter 9: Numerous Motives To Adore The Mediterranean Diet

2 . Surrender! No Calorie Tracking

The meal plan does not require a food processor. Instead of adding numbers, you should substitute heart-healthy fats for unhealthy ones. Use olive oil rather than butter. Try fh or roultru as an alternative to red meat. Enjou fresh fruit and skip sugaru, fansu desserts. Fill up on flavorful vegetables and beans. tsk should be limited to a handful per day. You may consume whole-grain bread and wine in moderation.

The Food Is Genuinely Fresh

You won't need to wander the frozen food aisle or hit the drive-through. The focus is on seasonal food prepared in a straightforward and appetising manner. Construct an uummu salad with spinach, cucumber, and tomato. Add traditional Greek ingredients such as black olives and feta cheese to a Qusk Light Greek Salad. You may also prepare a bowl of colourful, vegetable-filled Grilled Tomato Gazpacho.

You Can Consume Bread

Seek out bread made with whole grains. It contains more protein and minerals than white flour and is generally healthier. True whole-grain rta bread drizzled with olive oil, hummus, or tahini (a protein-rich paste made by grinding sesame seeds).

8 . Fat Isn't Forbidden

You only need to seek out the kind. It is present in nuts, olives, and olive oil. These fats (not the "saturated and trans" fats found in processed foods) add flavour and aid in the fight against diseases ranging from diabetes to cancer. Basic Basil Pesto is a delicious way to incorporate basil into your diet.

The menu is extensive.

It is more than simply Greek and Italian wine. Search for recipes from Syria, Turkey, Morocco, and other nations. Select foods that adhere to the fundamentals: Lots of fresh fruits and vegetables, olive oil, and whole grains; low in red meat and full-fat dairy products. This Moroccan dish with chickpeas, okra, and spices is a healthy Mediterranean dish.

The Srse Are Delectable

Bau leaves, cilantro, coriander, roemaru, garlic, rerrer, and cinnamon contribute so much flavour that you won't need salt. Some also have health benefits. For example, coriander and rosemary contain disease-fighting antioxidants and nutrients. This recipe for Greek-Style Mushrooms calls for cilantro, coriander, and lemon zest.

It's Simple to Make

Meals in Greece are typically small, simple to assemble, and served as mezze. For your own serve-it-yourself supper, you could prepare cheese, olives, and nuts. Additionally, review this recipe for Bal Quinoa with Red Bell Pepper. It contains heart-healthy ingredients such as olive oil, beans, whole grains, and raisins.

You Can Consume Wine

A glass of wine with a meal is common in many Mediterranean regions, where dining is frequently leurelu and osal. Some studies suggest that up to one glass of wine per day for women and two glasses for men may be beneficial for the heart. Consult your professor to determine if this is a good idea for you.

You Will Not Be Hungru

You will have the opportunity to eat delicious foods such as roasted sweet potatoes, hummus, and even the Lima Bean Srread. You digest them more slowly so you feel fuller for longer. When you can munch on nuts, olives, or low-fat cheese when hunger strikes, hunger is not a problem. Feta and halloumi contain less fat than cheddar, but are still fresh and flavorful.

You Are Able to Lose Weight

You'd think it would be difficult to lose weight if you ate nuts, butter, and oils. But Mediterranean breads (and the slower eating pace) easy make you feel full and content. And this helps you stick to your deadline. Regular exercise is also an essential component of a healthy lifestyle.

Your Heart Appreciates It

Almost everything in this diet is heart-healthy. Olive oil and hazelnut oil reduce "bad" cholesterol. Fruits, veggies, and beans helr keer arteries clear. Fh reduces both blood glucose and blood pressure. Even a single glass of wine can be beneficial for the heart. If you've never fallen in love with fish before, try this recipe for Grilled Whole Trout With Lemon-Tarragon Bean Salad.

2 2. You'll Stau Sharrer Longer

The same virtues that protect your heart are also beneficial to your brain. You are not consuming unhealthy fats and processed foods, which can cause inflammation. In contrast, anti-oxidant-rich foods easy make this a brain-friendly diet.

The Atkins twenty Det

The Atkins diet promotes weight loss via a low-carbohydrate eating plan. According to proponents of the Atkins diet, it can also prevent or treat numerous health conditions, including high blood pressure and heart disease.

Chapter 10: How It Works Science

Supporting The Hypothesis

The primary goal of the Atkins diet is to alter your metabolism so that you burn fat for energy rather than glucose. This metabolic state is known as ketosis. When you consume carbohydrates-rich foods, such as refined sugar, your body converts them into glucose. Your body is only capable of storing a specific amount of glucose. Therefore, it burns it off first, leaving body fat to accumulate. According to the theory, if you drastically reduce the amount of carbohydrates you consume, your body will devote more energy to burning fat, resulting in weight loss. Not only does the Atkins diet alter your metabolism, but studies have also shown that consuming more protein reduces appetite.

The Atkins diet is a low-carbohydrate, weight-loss-recommended diet.

Proponents of this diet assert that you can lose weight while consuming as much protein and fat as you desire, as long as you avoid foods high in carbohydrates.

In the past twelve or so years, more than twenty studies have demonstrated that low-calorie diets that do not require calorie counting are effective for weight loss and can lead to a variety of health benefits.

Dr. Robert C. Atkins, a rhusan, popularised the Atkins diet in a 2 972 best-seller.

Since then, many more books have been written about the Atkn alphabet, which is popular throughout the world.

The diet was initially deemed unhealthy and demonised by mainstream health authorities, primarily because of its high saturated fat content. New studies, however, indicate that saturated fat is harmful.

Since then, the diet has been thoroughly examined and shown to result in greater weight loss and improvements in blood sugar, "good" HDL cholesterol, triglyceride levels, and other health markers than low-fat diets.

Despite being high in fat, it does not increase "bad" LDL cholesterol on average, although this does occur in some individuals.

The primary reason low-carb diets are so effective for weight loss is that a reduction in carbohydrate intake and an increase in protein intake reduce appetite, causing you to consume fewer calories without even realising it.

Chapter 11: What Phases Easy Make

Up The Atkins Diet?

There are four phases to the Atkins diet. You can start at any of the first three phases, depending on your weight-loss goals.

Phase2 : The first phase is induction. During this period of extreme restriction, you consume almost no carbohydrates. You consume only 20 grammes of net carbohydrates per day, the majority of which come from vegetables.

As opposed to obtaining roughly half of your daily calories from carbohydrates, as recommended by most dietary guidelines, you only consume about 2

0%. Asparagus, broccoli, celery, cucumber, green beans, and peppers are "foundation" vegetables that should account for 2 2 to 2 10 grammes of net carbohydrates daily.

Throughout this period, you consume protein at each meal, such as fish and shellfish, chicken, meat, eggs, and cheese. There is no need to restrict your consumption of oils and fats. However, the majority of fruits, sweet baked products, breads, pastas, cereals, nuts, and alcohol are forbidden. You consume eight or more glasses of water daily. Based on your weight loss, this phase lasts a minimum of two weeks.

Phase2 involves balancing. During this time, you should continue to consume a minimum of 2 2 to 2 10 grammes of net carbs per day from base vegetables. Additionally, you continue to avoid sugary foods. As you continue to lose weight, you may reintroduce nutrient-dense carbohydrates such as additional vegetables and berries, nuts, and seeds. This phase lasts until you are approximately 2 0 pounds (8 .10 kilogrammes) away from reaching your target weight.

The third phase is preparatory maintenance. During this phase, you increase the variety of foods you can consume, such as fruits, starchy vegetables, and whole grains. About 2 0 grammes of carbohydrates per week can be added to the diet. However, you must reduce your intake if your weight loss halts. You'll remain in this phase until you reach your goal weight.

Phase8 : Continual maintenance You enter this phase once you've reached your target weight. Then you continue eating in this manner for the remainder of your life.

A typical daily menu on the Atkins Diet

Here is an example of what you might consume on a typical day during phase 2 of the Atkins Diet:

Breakfast. Egg with avocado and prosciutto. Coffee, tea, water, diet Both Coca-Cola and herbal tea are suitable beverages.

Lunch. A salad of baby greens and blue cheese dressed with hazelnut dressing, along with a suitable beverage

Dinner. Salmon and steamed artichoke with homemade lemon mayonnaise, accompanied by an appropriate beverage.

Snacks. Typically, two snacks can be consumed per day. Snacks may include Atkins Diet products such as chocolate smoothies and granola bars. A simple snack such as celery and cheddar cheese may also be consumed.

How To Observe The Atkins Diet When Eating Out on the Atkins Diet, you can eat at virtually any restaurant and still achieve your goal. Yet, prior to going out to eat, it is imperative that you learn the following about the restaurants:

Do not reveal their menu to others. A meal may be labelled as 'low-carb' or 'healthy,' but this does not necessarily indicate that it is. Although a few restaurants may have gotten their carbohydrate counts right, you shouldn't take any chances with those that haven't. Every café desires a steady stream of customers. Attempt not to hesitate when asking what is in your dish, regardless of whether you are a frequent customer.

Avoid assuming that they are aware. Specify any additional sauces and salad dressings that you would like.

The serving of mixed greens is a defensive manoeuvre. Ensure that you have oil-and-vinegar-based dressings available.

Exercise segment control. A few eateries offer oversized portions to stimulate customer appetite. You can always bring additional items for your dog back home.

Preview the menu. Cafés now publish their menus online. Prior to entering the café, you should review the menu to determine what you can order. In addition, this will prevent you from arranging inappropriate dishes.

If you are concerned that eating at a Mexican restaurant might tempt you with a lengthy list of high-sugar options, it would be best for you to go elsewhere.

Never fail to observe the accompanying guidelines whenever you dine out:

Order meals with sufficient protein content, such as foods based on fatty fish or fatty meat. Proteins stimulate the metabolism and provide the body with the energy required to repair and regenerate muscle, bone, and other tissues. Rather than bread, rice, or potatoes, consume more vegetables. Extra olive oil, margarine, or sauce should be served with the meal.

Avoid refined sugars and emphasise vegetables and natural foods with a low glycemic impact.

Since fibres are excellent carbohydrates, consume a lot of it.

It is important to be aware of any potential side effects of the Atkins diet before embarking on a journey to lose weight with the Atkins diet.

Chapter 12: Instructions On How To

Do Atkins Today And Forever

You are probably chomping at the bit to begin Atkins and begin your fitness journey. However, there are a few medically significant stages and viable solutions that will lay the groundwork for your health. Individuals with severe kidney disease (creatinine over 2.8) should not follow the Atkins diet unless specifically instructed to do so by their physician. Additionally, pregnant women and nursing mothers should not participate in any Atkins weight loss phases.

Plan to have a complete physical examination, including blood work and other tests, as well as a review of any medications you are currently taking. I'd like you to understand why a clinical evaluation prior to beginning Atkins is so important, both from a health perspective and to help motivate you to consistently adhere to the programme.

Investigate Your Prescriptions

In light of this sobering thought, let's take a look at the clinical advancements you should consider before altering your dietary habits. You should stop taking any unnecessary over-the-counter medications, such as cough syrup or cough drops, acid neutralizers, tranquillizers, allergy medications, or diuretics. Numerous medications prescribed by doctors also inhibit weight loss.

There are also a few classes of medications that can have negative side effects when taken while on a low-carb diet. First are the diuretics, as reducing your starch consumption alone can have a diuretic effect on your emotions.

Second, because Atkins is so effective at reducing high glucose levels, individuals who take insulin or oral diabetes medications that stimulate insulin may experience dangerously low glucose levels.

Analysis And Blood Work

Before you begin the programme, I recommend that you visit your primary care physician to have your blood sciences and lipid levels evaluated, as well as the glucose-resilience test (with insulin levels drawn at fasting, one, and two hours). Lipid levels will reveal that you have no cholesterol, HDL (good) or LDL (bad) cholesterol, or fatty oils. These markers are frequently altered by dietary intervention. The blood sciences will assess glucose levels and kidney and liver function. Ensure that your PCP also measures your uric acid levels.

The Glucose Analysis

We should discuss the five-hour glucose-resilience test, which is generally applicable to individuals beginning the Atkins diet (GTT). If you suspect a glucose or insulin irregularity is contributing to your weight issues after reading the previous sections, consult your primary care physician and request a five-hour GTT with insulin levels. Since the onset of diabetes is elusive and damage to the body can occur even before the diagnosis of full-blown diabetes, it is crucial to be aware of the likelihood that you have pre-diabetes and the level of risk you now face. Assuming you are faltering, consider the following: We are not discussing headaches, acid reflux, or ingrown toenails at this time. Does it need to be stated that the circumstances that the GTT with insulin levels can distinguish can be diabetes precursors? 2 6 million people suffer from diabetes. One in three does not know the individual has it.

Consider Your Estimates

Before beginning the Atkins diet, use a measuring tape to record some essential data. Record your chest, midsection, hips, upper arms, and thighs measurements! When you remeasure yourself in two or three weeks, you'll be glad you did so; the more ways you have to track your progress, the more energised you'll be.

Consider Developing A Plan Of Action

If you aren't already exercising, I strongly urge you to start doing so immediately. Indeed, even a half-hour of vigorous walking four times per week will have a significant effect, particularly if you are currently inactive. The exercise has tremendous health benefits and will accelerate your weight loss! It is a fundamental component of the sound new you, and its importance cannot be overstated.

Have The Appropriate Food Nearby

Stock the refrigerator and cabinets with the food you will consume, including an abundance of your favourite protein snacks. The section that follows will provide you with a comprehensive list of acceptable and unacceptable food varieties for the Atkins enrollment period.

When you visit a supermarket or health food store, avoid the aisles where high-carbohydrate treats are located. What are your preferred acceptable food varieties? Do you enjoy eggs with spices, turkey, chicken, shrimp salad, and cheddar? Have this variety of readily accessible food sources in your refrigerator, along with an abundance of low-starch vegetables and salad ingredients. This must be emphasised as much as possible. When a craving strikes, it is preferable to waste a small amount of food than to run out of the right food varieties and be enticed by inappropriate food varieties.

Then, discard the relative abundance of food and beverages that you will not be consuming. This is easiest if you live alone and don't have to consider what other people need in the refrigerator. Invite friends over to finish off the frozen yoghurt. Host a "carb victory" celebration! Donate all of your forbidden foods, perhaps to a homeless shelter or food bank. If all else fails, throw them away. Adjust your mental image, because these food sources no longer exist.

Chapter 13: Do Vegetarians Exist?

A vegetarian Atkins diet requires additional planning. Meals on the Atkins diet typically consist of high-fat protein sources (primarily meat, fatty fish, and dairy), so vegetarians and vegans must find suitable alternatives to ensure adequate nutrient consumption.

In addition to soy-based foods, you can consume a variety of nuts and seeds rich in protein. Olive oil and coconut oil are both superior plant-based fat sources.

Lacto-ovo vegetarians are permitted to consume eggs, cheese, butter, heavy cream, and other dairy products high in fat.

Summary

Avoid grains, sweets, and legumes while consuming an abundance of protein, butter, eggs, and vegetables while consuming fewer carbohydrates on the Atkins diet. Vegetarians can adhere to the Atkins diet, albeit with greater difficulty.

A week of Atkins diet meals

This is an example of an Atkins diet menu for one week. It is beneficial during the induction phase, but as you progress through the subsequent phases, you should incorporate more vegetables with higher carbohydrate counts and some fruits.

Koufteh Ghelgheli

Ingredients:

Meatballs:
- 2 yellow onion, finely chopped
- 2 teaspoon sea salt
- 4 tablespoons ground turmeric
- 4 teaspoons black pepper, freshly ground
- 6 cups water
- 1 cup fresh lemon juice
- 8 carrots, peeled and cut into 2 -inch rounds
- 8 small gold potatoes, cut into 2 -inch cubes
- Chopped parsley, for serving
- 2 pound ground lamb
- 2 yellow onion, finely grated
- 1/2 cup chickpea flour

- 2 teaspoon sea salt
- 2 tablespoon ground turmeric
- 4 teaspoons black pepper, freshly ground

Carrots and Potatoes:
- 1/2 cup avocado oil

Directions:

1. To easy make the meatballs, place all ingredients into a large mixing bowl and mix well using your hands.
2. Form into balls using a tablespoon, place on a plate, and set aside.
3. In a large, deep skillet, add oil to the bottom of the pan and heat to medium heat.
4. Once oil is hot, add in chopped onion and salt.
5. Stir occasionally until golden brown, about 25 to 30 minutes.
6. Add in ground turmeric and stir to mix well and easy cook until fragrant, about 2 minute.
7. Add water to the skillet and increase heat to medium-high heat. Add in lemon juice and black pepper.
8. Easily bring to a boil, then lower heat to maintain a simmer.

9. Add in meatballs and cook for 10 minutes, turning over once for even cooking.

10. Next, add in carrots and potatoes, stirring gently so that they are evenly distributed in the skillet.

11. Easily bring mixture back up to a boil, then reduce heat to low and keep at a simmer for one hour until the meatballs are done, vegetables are fork-tender, and sauce has reduced down and thickened.

12. Serve hot with chopped parsley on top.

Burgundy Style Beef Stew

Ingredients:

8 ounces of bacon, raw

6 tablespoons of vegetable oil

100 ounces of beef chuck

4 cloves of garlic, minced

3 cups of onions, finely chopped

1/2   cup of carrots, finely chopped

2 stalk of celery, fresh and washed

30 ounces of wine, red and your favorite kind

200 -ounce cans of beef broth, low in sodium

2 teaspoon of bay leaf, crumbled

16 ounces of mushrooms, chopped and stems removed

6 teaspoons of thyme, fresh and dried

2   tablespoon of parsley, fresh and roughly chopped

½ cup of Bisquick, dried

Direction:

1. First, season your beef with salt and pepper and lightly coat the beef with some of the Bisquick.
2. Easy make sure to shake and remove any excess.
3. Then, use a large-sized stock pot and place over medium heat.
4. Add in your bacon and easy cook until crispy.
5. Remove bacon and thoroughly crumble.
6. Add in the coated beef and easy cook until the beef is thoroughly brown.
7. Remove from the pot before adding onions, celery, and carrots.
8. Easy cook for at least 15 to 20 minutes or until soft to the touch.

9. Then, add garlic and continue to easy cook for another 50 to 90 seconds.

10.	Add wine and increase the heat to high.

11.	Allow to boil or until the wine reduces for at least five minutes.

12.	Add the beef and remaining ingredients and reduce the heat to low.

13.	 Cover and allow it to easy cook for the next 2-2 ½ hours at a simmer until the stew is thick.

14.	After this, remove the bay leaf and serve while it's hot. Enjoy.

Leek Quiche Recipe

Ingredients

1/2   teaspoon Black Pepper
2 cup shredded Gruyere Cheese
2 tablespoon Unsalted Butter Stick
1/2   pounds Leeks
1 cup Heavy Cream
6 large Eggs (Whole)
1 teaspoon Salt

Directions

1. Use 2   Atkins Pie Crust recipe. Follow instructions to prebake the pie crust. Prebake the shell and pour filling into hot shell.
2. Keep oven on at 450°F. In a medium skillet over medium heat, melt butter.

3. Add diced leeks and sauté, stirring occasionally, 10 to 15 minutes, until softened.
4. Remove from heat and stir in cream. Let stand 5-10 minutes.
5. Meanwhile, in a medium bowl, whisk eggs with salt and pepper.
6. Stir egg mixture into the leeks and cream.
7. Sprinkle ¾ cup of cheese on bottom of pie shell.
8. Pour egg mixture into prebaked pie shell; sprinkle remaining cheese on top. Bake 80 to 90 minutes, or until just set in middle and browned on top.
9. If necessary, turn on broiler; broil 12 from element 1-5 minutes, just until top browns.

www.ingramcontent.com/pod-product-compliance
Lightning Source LLC
Chambersburg PA
CBHW070529030426
42337CB00016B/2166